DEADLY INFECTIONS AND DISEASES

Discover deadly infections and diseases

on time before it kills

Healthy lifestyle is better than
deficiency, stay active and healthy

Dr Ben JAPHETH

Table of Contents:

- ANTIBIOTICS TREATMENT FOR
  BACTERIA INFECTIONS

- BEST ANTIBIOTICS DRUGS FOR FEVER
- BEST ANTIBIOTIC DRUGS FOR COUGH

Chapter 2

VIRAL INFECTIONS:

- PREVENTION AGAINST VIRAL INFECTIONS

- TREATMENT FOR VIRAL INFECTIONS

Chapter 3

FUNGAL INFECTIONS:

Chapter 4

WAYS TO IDENTIFY CANCER AND PREVENTION:

Chapter 5

WAYS TO IDENTIFY KIDNEY DISEASE AND PREVENTION:

Chapter 6

Chapter 7

WAYS TO IDENTIFY HIV INFECTION AND PREVENTION

Chapter 8

CAUSE FOR HIGH BLOOD PRESSURE AND TREATMENTS

- FOOD AND FRUIT THAT HELPS TO REDUCE HIGH BLOOD PRESSURE

- EXERCISE FOR HIGH BLOOD PRESSURE: Staying Active and Healthy

INTRODUCTION

Personal Health Care Prioritizing tone-Care for a Better Life particular health care is an essential aspect of our lives that's frequently neglected. With busy schedules and constant distractions, taking care of our internal and physical well-being can come grueling .

Still, prioritizing tone-care is pivotal to lead a happy and fulfilling life.
The first step in taking care of oneself is to maintain a healthy life by consuming a balanced diet and exercising regularly.

A balanced diet should include all food groups, similar to fruits, vegetables, grains, and proteins, to ensure that our bodies are getting all the necessary nutrients.

Exercise should also be incorporated into our diurnal routine, as it not only improves physical health but also boosts internal health.

According to a study published in the Journal of Psychiatric Research, regular exercise reduces anxiety and depression symptoms, increases tone-regard, and promotes better sleep. piecemeal from a healthy life, it's also essential to take care of our internal well- being.

Mental health issues, similar to depression and anxiety, have come increasingly common in moment's society.

Regular tone-check-sways can help us identify any signs of poor internal health and seek professional help when necessary. One effective system to take care of our internal health is by rehearsing awareness ways, similar as contemplation and deep breathing exercises.

A study by the National Center for Biotechnology Information set up that awareness-grounded stress reduction programs were effective in reducing stress, anxiety, and depression symptoms.

In addition to maintaining a healthy life and internal well-being, physical check-ups should also be a precedent.

Regular check-ups, similar to blood pressure and cholesterol tests, can help identify any implicit health problems at an early stage. Also, women should get regular Pap tests and mammograms, while men should get prostate examinations.

These wireworks are critical in detecting any signs of cancer or other ails at the foremost stage. Sleep is another aspect of particular health care that's frequently overlooked. Getting enough sleep is essential in maintaining good overall health and well-being.

According to the Centers for Disease Control and Prevention, grown-ups should aim for at least seven hours of sleep each night.

Lack of sleep can lead to colorful health issues, similar as mood swings, dropped cognitive function, and weakened impunity.
Taking care of one's particular health isn't only pivotal for physical and internal well-being but also leads to positive issues in other areas of life. For example, better health can lead to increased work productivity and creativity, better connections with musketeers and family, and a better quality of life overall. In conclusion, particular health care should be a top priority for individualities.

By prioritizing tone- care through maintaining a healthy life, taking care of internal and emotional well-being, getting regular physical check-ups, and getting enough sleep, individuals can lead happy and fulfilling lives.

IDENTIFY CONTAGIOUS CONDITIONS IN THE BODY

Infections are a broad order of ails that can be caused by a variety of pathogenic microorganisms similar as bacteria, contagions, fungi, and spongers.

They can range from mild, tone-limiting ails to severe, life-changing conditions. relating different types of infections is pivotal in determining the applicable treatment and precluding the spread of the infection. Then we bandy the most common types of infections and how you can identify them.

Chapter 1

Bacterial Infections:

Bacteria are unicellular microorganisms that can lead to a wide range of infections. The most common types of bacterial infections include streptococcal pharyngitis(strep throat), urinary tract infections, skin infections similar to impetigo and cellulitis, and bacterial pneumonia.

Generally, bacterial infections beget symptoms similar as fever, chills, coughing, sore throat, and fatigue. To identify bacterial infections, laboratory tests similar to blood societies, crack societies, and foam societies are used. The laboratory tests can help to insulate the specific type of bacteria causing the infection and also guide the selection of antibiotics for treatment.

<u>FORESTALLMENT AGAINST BACTERIA INFECTIONS</u>

Bacterial infections are caused by the growth and reduplication of dangerous bacteria within the body. These infections can lead to serious health problems if not treated duly. Still, there are several ways that can be taken to help bacterial infections.

The first step in precluding bacterial infections is to maintain good hygiene.

This includes washing your hands constantly with cleaner and warm water, especially after using the restroom or handling raw foods. It's also important to keep your surroundings clean and tidy.

Regularly drawing shells similar as countertops, door handles, and restroom institutions can help the spread of dangerous bacteria.

Another important step in precluding bacterial infections is to exercise safe food handling ways.

This includes cooking foods completely to kill dangerous bacteria, storing foods at the proper temperature, and avoiding cross-contamination by keeping raw flesh separate from other foods.

Eating a balanced diet that includes plenty of fruits and vegetables can also help strengthen the vulnerable system, making it easier for the body to fight off infections.

In addition to these introductory ways, there are several specific measures that can be taken to help bacterial infections.

For illustration, getting vaccinated against certain bacteria similar to pneumococcus and meningococcus can give protection against serious infections. Also, rehearsing safe coitus and using condoms can help the spread of sexually transmitted bacteria similar to

Chlamydia and gonorrhea. One of the most effective ways to help bacterial infections is through the use of antibiotics. Still, it's important to use these specifics only when necessary and to follow the specified lozenge and duration.

Overuse or abuse of antibiotics can lead to the development of antibiotic-resistant bacteria, which can be much more delicate to treat.

In conclusion, precluding bacterial infections requires a combination of introductory hygiene practices, safe food handling ways, healthy life choices, and specific measures similar to vaccination and antibiotic use.

By taking this way, we can reduce the threat of bacterial infections and cover our health and well- being.

Citations

(2021, February 15). precludingInfections. https//www.cdc.gov/infection control/prevent-infections/prevention.html

2. World Health Organization.(2017, January).
Health Topics Antibiotic Resistance. https//www.who.int/newsroom/fact-sheets/detail/antibiotic- resistance.

ANTIBIOTICS TREATMENT FOR BACTERIA

Antibiotics medicines have been one of the topmost discoveries in medical history. These medicines are used primarily in the treatment of bacterial infections and are responsible for saving millions of lives since their discovery in the early 20th century. Antibiotics similar to penicillin, erythromycin, and amoxicillin are generally used to treat bacterial infections similar to strep throat, pneumonia, and urinary tract infections. Antibiotics work by either killing the bacteria or by reducing its capability to reproduce and spread.

When a person is sick with a bacterial infection, their body's vulnerable system has difficulty fighting off the dangerous bacteria. This is where antibiotics come by.

Antibiotics can be administered intravenously, orally, or topically depending on the type and inflexibility of the infection, and the type of antibiotic being used. Antibiotics come in different classes and can thus have different mechanisms of action, meaning that antibiotics are frequently specified based on the type of bacterial infection that's present.

Antibiotics have been necessary in treating numerous severe infections, reducing mortality rates vastly.

Still, antibiotics have seen expansive use, frequently unnecessarily, which has led to an increase in antibiotic resistance and a drop in their efficacy. Antibiotic resistance occurs when bacteria develop a resistance to the antibiotics intended to kill them.

This resistance can affect the development of superbugs' ' which are resistant to multiple antibiotics and can be extremely grueling and expensive to treat. It's thus pivotal that antibiotics are used judiciously and only when necessary to help antibiotic resistance.

 When antibiotics are specified, it's essential to cleave to the specified lozenge and duration of treatment to help the development of resistance.

Also, cases shouldn't partake their antibiotics with others or stop taking them before the specified duration, as this can also contribute to antibiotic resistance.

It's also important to note that antibiotics only work against bacterial infections and are ineffective against viral infections, similar to the common cold wave or influenza.

Antibiotics can actually be dangerous when specified for viral infections because they can lead to implicit side-goods and contribute to antibiotic resistance. In similar cases, cases should follow treatment guidelines for viral infections, similar to rest and the use of over-the-counter specifics for symptom relief. In conclusion, antibiotics have been a precious tool for treating bacterial infections and have saved innumerous lives over the times.

Still, the overuse and abuse of antibiotics have led to the development of antibiotic resistance, which poses a significant public health problem.

It's thus pivotal that antibiotics are used judiciously and administered duly.

Cases should rigorously cleave to specified lozenge and duration, and be apprehensive that antibiotics don't treat viral infections. By following these guidelines, we can ensure that antibiotics remain an effective tool in treating bacterial infections for times to come.

BEST DRUGS FOR FEVER

Complications are one of the most common symptoms of ails, and while they're generally the result of an vulnerable response to an infection, they can also be caused by other factors similar as medicine responses and heat- related incidents. Anyhow, complications can leave individuals feeling relatively uncomfortable, and in some cases, they may indeed reach dangerous situations if left undressed. For that reason, there are a variety of

medicines available to treat fever. One of the most common medicines used to treat fever is acetaminophen.

Acetaminophen, also known as paracetamol, is a pain reliever and fever reducer that works by blocking the product of certain chemicals in the body that beget fever and inflammation. While acetaminophen is available over the counter, it's important to be apprehensive of the recommended lozenge and any implicit side goods. For illustration, taking too important acetaminophen can beget liver damage, and it can be dangerous for individuals who have certain medical conditions similar to liver complaints. Another popular medicine used to treat fever is ibuprofen. Ibuprofen is a non-steroidal anti-inflammatory medicine(NSAID) that works by reducing inflammation in the body. In addition to reducing complications, ibuprofen is also effective in treating mild to moderate pain, similar to headaches and toothaches. Like acetaminophen, ibuprofen is available over the counter, but it can have side effects similar to stomach derangement and increased threat of bleeding.

It's important to note that children under the age of six months shouldn't be given ibuprofen, and individualities with certain medical conditions should also avoid taking it. As with any drug, it's important to consult with a healthcare provider before taking fever- reducing medicines.

Some individuals may have medical conditions or be taking other specifics that could interact with fever- reducing medicines, and as a result, increase the threat of side goods.

Also, while fever- reducing medicines can give relief from fever- related symptoms, it's important to remember that they don't cure the beginning condition, and in some cases, they may indeed mask important symptoms.

For that reason, it's important to continue covering symptoms, and seek medical attention if they persist or worsen.

While acetaminophen and ibuprofen are two of the most generally used medicines for fever, there are other medicines and combinations of medicines that may be specified depending on the situation.

For illustration, croakers may define a combination of acetaminophen and an NSAID, or they may define tradition- strength pain relievers and anti-inflammatory medicines.

Each situation and existence is unique, and the course of treatment will depend on a variety of factors similar as underpinning conditions and inflexibility of symptoms. In addition to drugs, there are other ways individualities can take to help reduce fever- related symptoms.

For illustration, getting plenty of rest, staying doused , and keeping the terrain cool can all help palliate discomfort.

It's also important to avoid emphatic exertion and alcohol consumption, as these can increase the threat of dehumidification and complicate fever- related symptoms.

In conclusion, fever- reducing medicines similar to acetaminophen and ibuprofen can give relief from fever- related symptoms, but it's important to consult with a healthcare provider and follow recommended tablets to avoid implicit side effects. While drugs can be helpful, it's also important to flash back that they don't cure the beginning condition and to continue covering symptoms.

Also, individualities should take a way to watch for themselves and promote mending similar to getting plenty of rest and staying doused .

Eventually, a multifaceted approach to fever treatment that includes medical guidance and tone- care can lead to better issues and relief from discomfort.

Cough is a kickback action that helps clear mucus and foreign substances from the lungs and airways.

It serves as a pivotal defense medium for our body. Still, a patient and troubling cough can be extremely perverse and uncomfortable, leading to sleep disturbances, fatigue, and reduced quality of life.

Thus, treating cough effectively is essential, and the use of the right drug can give characteristic relief. In this essay, we will bandy the stylish medicines for cough and their mechanisms of action. The choice of medicines for cough depends largely on the underpinning cause.

Coughs in general terms can be classified as productive ornon-productive.

Productive coughs, generally known as phlegmy or chesty coughs, produce mucus or numbness and are caused by infections like the common cold wave, flu, or bronchitis.

On the other hand,non-productive, also known as dry or tickly coughs, are caused by annoyances, allergens, and other factors that beget inflammation in the airways, leading to the cough kickback.

One of the most effective medicines for a productive cough is guaifenesin, generally retailed under the brand name Mucinex. It's an expectorant that works by lacing the mucus in the airways, making it easier to cough up.

A meta- analysis of six randomized controlled trials established that guaifenesin was effective in reducing cough frequency and perfecting foam salivation in cases with acute respiratory tract infections.

The experimenters concluded that guaifenesin could be a precious treatment option for cough in these

Chapter 2

Viral Infections

Contagions are contagious agents that bear a host cell to replicate. Some common viral infections include the common cold wave, influenza, gastroenteritis(stomach flu), and viral hepatitis. Different contagions can beget different symptoms, but common clinical instantiations of viral infections include fever, headache, watery nose, cough, sore throat, and fatigue.

To identify viral infections, laboratory tests similar to viral culture, polymerase chain response(PCR), and serology are performed. Viral culture involves taking a sample of body fluid, similar to blood or foam, and growing the contagion in a culture dish. PCR is a sensitive test that can decry contagions grounded on their inheritable material. In discrepancy, serology tests determine whether a case has preliminarily been exposed to a particular contagion by detecting the presence of antibodies in their blood.

FORESTALLMENT AGAINST VIRAL INFECTIONS

Contagious are bitsy organisms that can beget colorful health problems in humans. Viral infections are a common consequence of these microorganisms.

Contagions enter a host cell and take over the cell's ministry to replicate, reproduce, and foray other host cells. Viral infections are spread through different ways, similar as physical contact, defiled food or water, and through the air. Thus, to help prevent viral infections, it's essential to maintain particular hygiene, follow preventative measures, and get vaccinated. One of the most effective ways to help viral infections is to maintain particular hygiene.

particular hygiene refers to the colorful practices that people follow to keep themselves clean and maintain health. These practices include washing hands with cleaner and water constantly, covering the mouth and nose while coughing or sneezing, and taking a bath or shower regularly.

Washing hands with cleaner and water is the most effective way to help viral infections as it eliminates contagions that may have been picked up from defiled shells. By washing hands with cleaner and water, the contagions aren't only removed from the hands, but it also destroys them.
A study conducted by the Centers for Disease Control and Prevention(CDC) showed that handwashing with cleaner and water reduced respiratory infections by 16-21 **(Gould,C.V et al, 2020) **. Another way to help viral infections is by following preventative measures.

These measures aim to minimize contact with contagions and reduce the spread of infections.

preventative measures include avoiding close contact with people who are sick, not touching the eyes, nose, or mouth without washing hands first, and disinfecting constantly touched objects and shells. These measures also include wearing nose masks and social distancing, which are veritably important during this COVID- 19 epidemic. Social distancing, for illustration, reduces direct physical contact, therefore precluding the spread of contagions through driblets. A study by Morawska,L. etal.,(2020) supported the effectiveness of social distancing in reducing the transmission of COVID- 19--- a new coronavirus that has spread across the globe fleetly. Incipiently, getting vaccinated is a veritably pivotal way to help viral infections. Vaccines are medical products that work by stimulating the vulnerable system to produce antibodies that cover against specific viral infections. Vaccines help individualities from getting infected, lower the inflexibility of the complaint, and reduce the threat of severe complications.

Vaccines have been used to successfully help viral infections similar to Polio, Measles, Mumps, Rubella, Smallpox, and Hepatitis B, among others. Vaccines have also shown a high rate of efficacy in guarding against contagions like influenza. It's veritably important to punctuate that vaccines aren't only salutary to the vaccinated person but also to the society as a whole. When a large chance of the population is vaccinated, this conception of community impunity or herd impunity is achieved, where indeed those who aren't vaccinated are defended from the viral infections.

In conclusion, viral infections present a significant health challenge encyclopedically. Prevention of viral infections begins with maintaining particular hygiene, following preventative measures similar as social distancing and disinfection, and getting vaccinated.

particular hygiene, as simple as handwashing, has shown to be veritably effective in reducing the chances of infections. preventative measures similar as social distancing and wearing masks also play a vital part in reducing the spread of contagions. Vaccines are also effective in precluding viral infections and are pivotal for the individual and Public health.

It's important to always follow these forestallment measures, especially in this age of the COVID- 19 epidemic.

TREATMENT FOR VIRAL INFECTIONS

Viral infections are caused by the irruption of contagions into mortal bodies and can lead to several ails, including the common cold wave, flu, and indeed some types of cancer. Treating viral infections is frequently delicate because there are limited antiviral specifics, and developing vaccines for viral infections is a time-consuming process. Still, colorful strategies can be used to manage viral infections.

This essay will bandy the treatment for viral infections, including antiviral specifics, vaccines, and natural remedies.

Antiviral specifics Antiviral specifics are the primary treatment for viral infections. Antiviral medicines work by blocking the contagion's capability to replicate inside a host cell, thereby reducing complaint inflexibility and precluding the spread of infection. There are several antiviral specifics available that are effective for treating viral infections similar to HIV, herpes, influenza and hepatitis. For illustration, acyclovir is a medicine used to treat herpes simplex contagion, and tenofovir is used to treat HIV infection. It's essential to note that not all viral infections can be treated with antiviral specifics.

Vaccines Vaccines are an effective way to help viral infections. Vaccines work through stimulating the vulnerable system to develop impunity to a specific contagion. Vaccines work by exposing the body to a weakened or inactive form of the contagion, which triggers the vulnerable system to produce antibodies against the contagion. This process of vaccination means that when the existent is exposed to the contagion, the vulnerable system can fefe and fight the contagion more effectively, precluding the development of a viral infection. Lately, the world has seen the development of several vaccines to combat the COVID-19 contagion, which has caused a global epidemic. Several vaccines, similar as Pfizer- BioNTech, Moderna, Johnson & Johnson, and AstraZeneca, have been authorized by nonsupervisory agencies worldwide for exigency use. These vaccines have been shown to be effective in precluding severe COVID- 19 infection and reducing COVID-19-related hospitalizations and deaths. Still, it's worth noting that vaccines aren't a guaranteed cure for viral infections and may not be effective for all contagions. Natural Remedies Several natural remedies claim to treat viral infections. These remedies include factory- grounded products similar to echinacea and elderberry, which are said to help boost the vulnerable system, and honey and garlic, which have antimicrobial parcels. There are also certain vitamins, similar as vitamin C, and minerals, similar as zinc, that are believed to help reduce the inflexibility and duration of viral infections. Still, the use of natural remedies for viral infections is largely untested scientifically. As a result, it's unclear whether these remedies are effective against viral infections or not. Conclusion Viral infections can beget severe ails and pose a significant threat to public health. The treatment of viral infections includes antiviral specifics, vaccines, and natural remedies. Antiviral specifics are effective for treating some viral infections, while vaccines can be used to help viral infections. Natural remedies may help manage the symptoms of viral infections, but their effectiveness remains untested scientifically.

Healthcare providers should readily diagnose viral infections and recommend the applicable treatment strategy for their cases. Citations 1. Focosi D et al. Antiviral remedy of mortal papillomavirus. World journal of virology. 2012; 1(1) 9 – 19. doi 10.5501/wjv.v1.i1.9 2. Polack,F.P et al. New England Journal of Medicine. DOI10.1056/ NEJMoa2034577

Chapter 3

Fungal Infections

Fungi are a different group of microorganisms that can beget a variety of infections in humans. Common fungal infections include thrush(oral candidiasis), ringworm, athlete's bottom, and vaginal incentive infections. Symptoms of fungal infections can include itching, greenishness, scaling, and vexation of the affected area. To identify fungal infections, a variety of laboratory tests are available, including societies and bitsy examination of the affected towel. Tests similar to serology and PCR can also be used to describe fungal infections in some cases. Parasitic Infections spongers are organisms that depend on a host organism to survive. They can beget a range of infections, including malaria, giardiasis,toxoplasmosis,and cryptosporidiosis.

Symptoms of parasitic infections may vary depending on the type of sponger and can include fever, diarrhea, abdominal pain, and skin rashes. To diagnose parasitic infections, a variety of laboratory tests similar as blood tests, coprolite tests, and imaging tests may be used. In some cases, a vivisection may be necessary to identify the sponger in the affected towel. In conclusion, infections can be caused by a variety of microorganisms, including bacteria, contagions, fungi, and spongers. relating the type of infection is essential in determining the applicable treatment and precluding the spread of the infection. Laboratory tests similar to societies, serology, and PCR can be used to diagnose different types of infections. It's pivotal to seek medical attention if you suspect you have an infection, as early identification and treatment can help speed your recovery and help further complications. --- workshop Cited - getaway,T.T., & Shaddock,J.H.(2020). contagious conditions. In StatPearls(Internet). StatPearls Publishing. - Crawford,J.M.(2019). Practical approach to contagious conditions. Lippincott Williams & Wilkins.

FORESTALLMENT AGAINST FUNGAL INFECTION

Fungi are eukaryotic organisms that can beget infections in humans. The most common fungal infections include candidiasis, ringworms, and aspergillosis, among others. Fungal infections can affect different corridors of the body, including the skin, lungs, and nails. Prevention of fungal infections involves measures that reduce the threat of contracting them. In this essay, I'll bandy some of the forestallment measures to prevent fungal infections. originally, good particular hygiene is critical in precluding fungal infections. Maintaining particular hygiene keeps the skin dry and clean, discouraging the growth and spread of fungi. Fungi thrive in warm and wettish surroundings, especially in sweaty areas of the body, similar to the armpits, groin, and bases. Thus, it's essential to take a bath at least once a day, especially after sharing in conditioning that makes one sweat. After a shower, one should dry their body completely, particularly in the crowds of the skin, where fungi tend to grow. Drying the body helps to help the growth and spread of fungi. Also, one should avoid wearing tight- befitting apparel as they can promote the accumulation of sweat, creating a conducive terrain for fungi growth. Secondly, maintaining a healthy life can also help help fungal infections. A healthy diet that's rich in vitamins and minerals helps to boost the vulnerable system, reducing the threat of fungal infections. Foods similar to garlic, gusto, and turmeric have antifungal parcels, which also help to keep fungal infections at bay. Regular exercise also helps to ameliorate the vulnerable system, reduce stress, and enhance blood rotation, which helps to help fungal infections. individuals with underpinning medical conditions similar to diabetes should manage their conditions well to help fungal infections. Diabetes cases are at an advanced threat of developing fungal infections since high blood sugar situations increase the threat of infections and decelerate down the mending process.

Also, immunocompromised individuals should take measures to reduce their threat of fungal infections. These individualities include HIV/ AIDS cases, organ transplant donors, and cancer cases entering chemotherapy. Thirdly, taking caution when engaging in out-of-door conditioning can also help fungal infections. Fungi are present in the terrain and can fluently infect individuals engaged in out-of-door conditioning similar to hiking, gardening, or playing in the soil. It's important to wear defensive gear similar to gloves and shoes when sharing similar conditioning. Also, one should avoid walking barefoot on defiled shells similar to public showers, locker apartments, and swimming pools. Fungi thrive in warm and wettish surroundings, making similar shells ideal breeding grounds.

Using antifungal maquillages or sprays also helps to help fungal infections. Incipiently, maintaining good oral hygiene is essential in precluding fungal infections.

The mouth is home to numerous microorganisms, including fungi. Poor oral hygiene increases the threat of developing fungal infections similar to oral thrush, which is caused by an incentive called candida. Thus, brushing teeth twice a day and using mouthwash helps to help fungal infections. Also, individuals with dentures should be careful when drawing them as they're also prone to fungal infections. It's important to clean them completely and store them in a clean and dry place to help fungal growth. In conclusion, forestallment of fungal infections involves measures that reduce the threat of contracting them. Good particular hygiene, maintaining a healthy life, taking caution when engaging in out-of-door conditioning, and maintaining good oral hygiene are some of the critical forestallment measures. By espousing these measures, individualities can significantly reduce their threat of developing fungal infections.

TREATMENT FOR FUNGAL INFECTIONS

Fungi are a different group of microorganisms that can beget a variety of infections in humans. Common fungal infections include thrush(oral candidiasis), ringworm, athlete's bottom, and vaginal incitement infections. Symptoms of fungal infections can include itching, greenness, scaling, and vexation of the affected area. To identify fungal infections, a variety of laboratory tests are available, including societies and bitty examination of the affected kerchief. Tests analogous as serology and PCR can also be used to describe fungal infections in some cases. Parasitic Infections freeloaders are organisms that depend on a host organism to survive. They can beget a range of infections, including malaria, giardiasis, toxoplasmosis, and cryptosporidiosis. Symptoms of parasitic infections may vary depending on the type of sponge and can include fever, diarrhea, abdominal pain, and skin rashes. To diagnose parasitic infections, a variety of laboratory tests analogous as blood tests, excreta tests, and imaging tests may be used. In some cases, a dissection may be necessary to identify the sponge in the affected kerchief. In conclusion, infections can be caused by a variety of microorganisms, including bacteria, contagions, fungi, and freeloaders. relating the type of infection is essential in determining the applicable treatment and preventing the spread of the infection. Laboratory tests analogous as societies, serology, and PCR can be used to diagnose different types of infections. It's vital to seek medical attention if you suspect you have an infection, as early identification and treatment can help speed your recovery and help further complications. --- factory Cited- flight,T.T., & Shaddock,J.H.(2020). contagious conditions. In StatPearls(Internet). StatPearls Publishing. - Crawford,J.M.(2019). Practical approach to contagious conditions. Lippincott Williams & Wilkins.

PREVENTION AGAINST FUNGAL INFECTIONS

Fungi are eukaryotic organisms that can beget infections in humans.
The most common fungal infections include candidiasis, ringworms, and aspergillosis, among others. Fungal infections can affect different corridors of the body, including the skin, lungs, and nails. Prevention of fungal infections involves measures that reduce the trouble of contracting them. In this essay, I will discuss some of the prevention measures to fungal infections. Firstly, good hygiene is critical in preventing fungal infections. Maintaining particular hygiene keeps the skin dry and clean, discouraging the growth and spread of fungi. Fungi thrive in warm and damp surroundings, especially

in sweaty areas of the body, analogous as the armpits, groin, and bases. Therefore, it's essential to take a bath at least once a day, especially after participating in exertion that makes one sweat. After a shower, one should dry their body fully, particularly in the crowds of the skin, where fungi tend to grow. Drying the body helps to help the growth and spread of fungi. Also, one should avoid wearing tight-befitting vestures as they can promote the accumulation of sweat, creating a conducive terrain for fungi growth. Secondly, maintaining a healthy life can also help help fungal infections. A healthy diet that is rich in vitamins and minerals helps to boost the vulnerable system, reducing the trouble of fungal infections. Foods analogous as garlic, ginger, and turmeric have antifungal parcels, which also help to keep fungal infections at bay. Regular exercise also helps to heal the vulnerable system, reduce stress, and enhance blood gyration, which helps to help fungal infections.

Individuals with bolstering medical conditions analogous to diabetes should manage their conditions well to help fungal infections. Diabetes cases are at an advanced trouble of developing fungal infections since high blood sugar situations increase the trouble of infections and break down the healing process.

Also, immunocompromised individuals should take measures to reduce their trouble with fungal infections. These individualities include HIV/ AIDS cases, organ transplant benefactors, and cancer cases entering chemotherapy. Thirdly, taking caution when engaging in out- of- door exertion can also help fungal infections. Fungi are present in the terrain and can easily infect individuals engaged in out- of- door exertion analogous as hiking, gardening, or playing in the soil. It's important to wear protective gear analogous to gloves and shoes when participating in analogous exertion. Also, one should avoid walking barefoot on defiled shells analogous to public showers, locker apartments, and swimming pools. Fungi thrive in warm and damp surroundings, making analogous shells ideal breeding grounds. Using antifungal maquillages or sprays also helps to help fungal infections. Initially, maintaining good oral hygiene is essential in preventing fungal infections.

The mouth is home to multitudinous microorganisms, including fungi. Poor oral hygiene increases the trouble of developing fungal infections analogous to oral thrush, which is caused by an incitement called candida. Therefore, brushing teeth twice a day and using mouthwash helps to help fungal infections.

Also, individuals with dentures should be careful when drawing them as they are also prone to fungal infections. It's important to clean them fully and store them in a clean and dry place to help fungal growth. In conclusion, prevention of fungal infections involves measures that reduce the trouble of contracting them.

Good hygiene, maintaining a healthy life, taking caution when engaging in out- of- door exertion, and maintaining good oral hygiene are some of the critical prevention measures. By espousing these measures, individualities can significantly reduce their trouble of developing fungal infections.

Chapter 4

WAYS TO IDENTIFY CANCER AND PREVENTION

Cancer, despite its adding frequency, remains one of the most delicate conditions to describe and treat. Cancer webbing programs and forestallment styles are reckoned upon heavily to reduce the prevalence of the complaint and ameliorate the issues for those affected. In this essay, we will examine the ways to identify cancer and forestallment. Relating cancer at an early stage is pivotal for prompt operation and effective treatment. Some relative approaches can identify cancer, including imaging studies like mammography or colonoscopy as well as blood tests, vivisection, and inheritable testing. The opinion of cancer is determined by multiple factors, including clinical findings, molecular tests, and imaging studies. colorful webbing measures are recommended for specific cancers. For illustration, the most common webbing test for bone cancer in ladies is mammography. This webbing tool has lowered the mortality rates of bone cancer by detecting early- stage complaints when it's utmost treatable. Screening with mammography is recommended every time or two beginning at age 50 times for utmost women. An analogous approach works for cervical cancer webbing, which involves a regular Pap smear. While webbing tools are an essential tool, it's vital to know your body so you can fend off any physical changes that are out of the ordinary. tone- examination for cancers like bone cancer is recommended regularly. Women are advised to check their guts at least once a month for any abnormal changes or lumps. Early discovery is essential, but taking preventative measures is just as important. variations in life can help colorful types of cancers. An unhealthy life, including unhealthy diets and lack of physical exertion, can increase your threat for cancer. substantiation has shown that regular physical exercise can reduce the prevalence of some cancers. The American Cancer Society recommends at least 150 twinkles of moderate exercise per week or 75 twinkles of vigorous exercise. A healthy diet that includes abundant factory foods, fiber, and limited beast products can help reduce the threat of developing numerous types of cancers. Some salutary considerations of early studies have shown a correlation between high sugar consumption and some cancers. Tobacco smoking remains the most preventable cause of cancer. The chemicals present in smoking tobacco can damage DNA and increase the threat of developing numerous types of cancers similar to lung, throat, and bladder. The simple answer is to quit smoking. Giving up smoking indeed for those who have smoked for decades reduces the threat of tobacco- associated cancer. Regular alcohol input has been associated with an advanced threat of developing liver, bone, and colon cancers. Smoking tobacco and drinking alcohol are leading causes for some types of cancers. It's recommended to limit both smoking and alcohol consumption.

It's essential to adopt the HPV vaccine to avoid the mortal papillomavirus(HPV) infection. HPV can beget cervical and anal cancer as well as some throat and lingo cancers.

The HPV vaccine is given to children aged 11- 12 times and is recommended in youthful grown-ups who nowadays entered the vaccine.

In addition to the below preventative measures, getting enough sleep and reducing stress can also help avoid cancer. Sleep privation and habitual stress can lead to diseases of the vulnerable system and increase inflammation, leading to cancer growth. So, getting a good night's sleep and reducing stress in your life can help cure cancer. In conclusion, treating cancer at an early stage is pivotal for prompt operation and effective treatment. colorful webbing measures are available, including, for illustration, mammography for bone cancer webbing.

TONE-CARE examination and life variations can also reduce the threat of cancer. Tobacco smoking and alcohol consumption are leading causes of some cancers, so avoiding them is imperative. The HPV vaccine is pivotal to help infections that can beget cervical and anal cancers. Getting enough sleep and reducing stress can also help cancer.

Chapter 5

WAYS TO IDENTIFY KIDNEY DISEASE AND PREVENTION

Order complaint is a potentially dangerous condition that can beget a variety of health problems. numerous people don't realize they've ordered a complaint until the complaint has progressed to a severe stage, and this can be a major problem for their health and well- being. In this essay, I'll describe ways to identify order complaints and ways one can take to help it from being in the first place. One of the most common ways to identify order complaints is through routine blood and urine tests. These tests can help to identify abnormalities in the blood or urine, which may indicate a problem with the feathers. Some of the most common abnormalities that may be detected include high situations of protein or blood in the urine, low situations of red blood cells, When these abnormalities are detected, a croaker

may order fresh tests to determine the cause and inflexibility of the order complaint. Another way to identify order complaints is through imaging tests similar to an ultrasound or CT checkup.

These tests can help to punctuate any structural abnormalities in the feathers and may be useful in relating the presence of order monuments, excrescences, or excrescences. In some cases, a order vivisection may also be used to diagnose order complaint. This involves taking a small sample of towel from the order and examining it under a microscope to look for signs of inflammation, scarring, or other abnormalities. Once an order complaint has been linked, there are several ways one can take to help it from progressing to a more severe stage.
One of the most important ways is to manage any beginning conditions that may be contributing to order complaints. This may involve controlling high blood pressure, managing diabetes, or treating infections that may be affecting the feathers.

Another important step in precluding order complaints is to maintain a healthy life. Eating a healthy, balanced diet can help to reduce the threat of developing conditions similar as high blood pressure and diabetes, which are contributing factors to the development of order complaint. Exercise is also important for maintaining overall health and may help to reduce the threat of developing order complaint. In addition to managing beginning conditions and maintaining a healthy life, there are several other way one can take to help order complaint. These include avoiding specifics and substances that may be dangerous to the feathers, similar as nonsteroidal anti-inflammatory medicines(NSAIDs) and illegal medicines. It's also important to stay doused and to avoid getting dehydrated, as this can put fresh strain on the feathers.

In conclusion, order complaints can be a serious and potentially life- hanging condition. Still, with early identification and proper operation, it's possible to help the complaint from progressing to a more severe stage. Routine blood and urine tests, along with imaging tests and order necropsies, can be used to identify order complaints.

Once the complaint has been linked, a way can be taken to manage beginning conditions, maintain a healthy life, and help further damage to the feathers. By taking these ways, individualities can reduce their threat of developing order complaints and ameliorate their overall health and well- being.

Chapter 6

WAYS TO IDENTIFY LIVER DISEASE AND PREVENTION

Liver complaint refers to a condition where your liver is damaged or bloodied. The liver is an important organ that helps in digestion, detoxification of the body, and synthesizing important proteins. The most common types of liver conditions are non-alcoholic adipose liver complaint(NAFLD), hepatitis, andcirrhosis.However, liver conditions can come life- hanging , If left undressed. Thus, it's important to identify and help liver complaints. In this essay, I'll outline colorful ways to identify liver complaints and explore preventative measures.

One of the most effective ways of relating liver complaint is through blood tests. Blood tests help to identify liver function by measuring the situations of specific enzymes and proteins. Some of the most generally measured enzymes include alanine aminotransferase(ALT) and aspartate aminotransferase(AST).

When the liver is damaged or inflamed, these enzymes are released into the bloodstream, leading to high situations in the blood. Blood tests are also used to measure the situations of bilirubin, a unheroic color responsible for hostility.

When the liver isn't performing correctly, bilirubin situations can come elevated, leading to hostility. In addition, blood tests can also descry the presence of antibodies that indicate hepatitis infection. piecemeal from blood tests, imaging tests are another way to identify liver complaint. Imaging tests include ultrasound, CT checkup, MRI, and elastography. These tests help to descry signs of complaint by revealing any abnormalities in the liver. For illustration, ultrasound helps to identify any changes in the liver's size or texture. also, CT reviews and MRI can identify any liver millions or excrescences. Elastography is a newer fashion that uses sound swells to measure the liver's stiffness. Stiffness is a measure of liver damage, and elastography scores can help to diagnose liver complaint. In addition to medical tests, there are also some visible symptoms that help to identify liver complaints.

One of the most common symptoms of liver complaint is hostility, a condition characterized by yellowing of the skin and eyes. Cases with liver complaints may also witness abdominal pain, extreme fatigue, and nausea. Bleeding or bruising fluently, loss of appetite, and swelling in the legs are some fresh symptoms associated with liver complaints.

Prevention of liver complaints is important to avoid the development of serious liver conditions. The following tips can help in the forestallment of liver complaint

1) Reduce alcohol input- Drinking too much alcohol can harm the liver. It's important to ensure that one's alcohol input doesn't exceed 1- 2 drinks per day.

2) Maintain a healthy weight-Non-alcoholic adipose liver complaint(NAFLD) is caused by the accumulation of fat in the liver. Maintaining a healthy weight is important in precluding NAFLD.

3) Stay doused - Drinking plenitude of water helps to flush out poisons from the liver, which is important in maintaining liver health.

4) Get vaccinated- Vaccines for hepatitis A and B can help cover against these infections, which can beget liver complaints.

5) Reduce exposure to poisons- Exposure to dangerous chemicals and drugs can damage the liver. It's important to follow proper safety guidelines when handling dangerous chemicals and to follow proper operation instructions for drugs. In conclusion, liver conditions can be grueling to diagnose and treat if not linked beforehand.

Blood tests, imaging tests, and visible symptoms similar to hostility can all help in the identification of liver complaints. preventative measures similar as reducing alcohol input, maintaining a healthy weight, staying doused , getting vaccinated, and reducing exposure to poisons can all help in the forestallment of liver complaints. Maintaining liver health is pivotal in precluding the development of serious liver conditions.

Chapter 7

WAYS TO IDENTIFY HIV INFECTION AND PREVENTION

Mortal Immunodeficiency Contagion(HIV) is a serious contagion that affects the vulnerable system, leading to weakened defenses against infections and other conditions. HIV is substantially transmitted through blood, semen, vaginal fluids, and bone milk. More specifically, HIV can be transmitted through sexual intercourse(anal, vaginal, or oral), participating needles, blood transfusions, and during gestation, parturition or breastfeeding. Knowing the signs and symptoms of HIV infection is pivotal because early discovery and treatment can significantly ameliorate patient issues. The common symptoms of HIV infection can vary from person to person and can be analogous to those of other viral infections, similar to flu or mononucleosis.

Some common symptoms of acute HIV infection include fever, headache, muscle pangs, fatigue, sore throat, blown lymph bumps, skin rash, and mouth blisters. These symptoms may develop within two to four weeks after a person has been infected with HIV and generally go down on their own.

Still, some people may not witness any symptoms at all during this early stage of the infection. After the original stage of acute infection, HIV can continue to damage the vulnerable system without causing any conspicuous symptoms.

It may take several times for symptoms of advanced HIV infection, also known as acquired immunodeficiency pattern(AIDS), to appear. These symptoms may include habitual diarrhea, fever, night sweats, unexplained weight loss, habitual fatigue, fungal infections, and certain types of cancer. Prevention of HIV infection is pivotal as there's still no cure for HIV.

It's important to exercise safe coitus, use condoms constantly and rightly, and get tested for HIV and other sexually transmitted infections regularly. People who fit medicines should always use clean needles and norway partake needles, hypes, or any other injection outfit. Likewise, HIV can also be averted through pre-exposure prophylaxis(PrEP), which involves taking HIV drugs daily to reduce the threat of HIV infection. Another important aspect of HIV forestallment is education and mindfulness. Educating people on how HIV is transmitted, how to cover themselves from it, and how to get tested for HIV can help reduce the spread of the contagion. HIV smirch and demarcation can also hamper HIV forestallment sweats.

People living with HIV may witness demarcation or fear of smirch, which can help them from penetrating medical care and telling their HIV status to mates. In conclusion, HIV remains a serious public health concern, and forestallment sweats are critical in controlling its spread. Feting the signs and symptoms of HIV infection can lead to early discovery and treatment, which can significantly ameliorate patient issues. Prevention styles, including safe coitus practices, PrEP, and education and mindfulness, can help reduce the transmission of HIV. It's important to continue to support people living with HIV and work towards reducing HIV smirch and demarcation within society.

Chapter 8

CAUSES OF HIGH BLOOD PRESSURE AND TREATMENT

High blood pressure, also known as hypertension, is a condition when the pressure in the highways is constantly elevated. Hypertension can lead to severe medical problems similar to heart failure, stroke, order complaint, and heart attack.

Millions of people worldwide are affected by high blood pressure, and the condition can remain undetected for a long time without showing any conspicuous signs or symptoms. In this essay, we will detail the causes of high blood pressure in detail.

One of the main causes of high blood pressure is an unhealthy life, including rotundity, physical inactivity, and an unhealthy diet. Rotundity increases the threat of hypertension because it puts redundant pressure on the heart, making it harder than usual to circulate blood throughout the body.

Also, physical inactivity and a diet low in whole grains, fruits, and vegetables, but high in sugar, sugar, and fat, can each contribute to hypertension. Another possible cause of high blood pressure is age and genetics. Blood pressure tends to increase with age, and individuals with a family history of hypertension are at an advanced threat of developing the condition. According to a study, genetics account for roughly 30- 50 of the variability in blood pressure, and individualities with a family history of hypertension have a two-fold increased threat of developing essential hypertension compared to those without a family history.

TREATMENT FOR HIGH BLOOD PRESSURE

High blood pressure, also known as hypertension, is a common medical condition. It can lead to colorful health complications if left undressed. According to the World Health Organization(WHO), high blood pressure is the leading cause of mortality worldwide, and it accounts for 7.5 million deaths annually encyclopedia ally. Fortunately, numerous treatments are available that can help treat high blood pressure. In this essay, we will explore some of the most common treatments available for high blood pressure. The Non-pharmacological treatment options for high blood pressure include life changes similar as modifying your diet, reducing swab input, losing weight, and adding physical exertion. Salutary approaches to stop hypertension(gusto) is one of the most popular diets that people with high blood pressure follow. It's low in swab, impregnated fat, and cholesterol but rich in fruits, vegetables, whole grains, and low- fat dairy products, and it has been shown to significantly reduce blood pressure situations.

Reducing swab input is another largely effective non-pharmacological approach to lower blood pressure. The American Heart Association recommends lower than 1500 milligrams of sodium per day for people with high blood pressure. This can be achieved by cooking fresh foods at home, avoiding reused foods, and checking the markers of packaged products to insure they're low in sodium. Engaging in regular physical exertion can also help lower blood pressure.
The American Heart Association recommends getting at least 150 twinkles of moderate- intensity exercise per week, or at least 75 twinkles of vigorous- intensity exercise per week. This can include conditioning similar to brisk walking, cycling, or swimming.

In addition to non-pharmacological treatments, several specifics are available to treat high blood pressure. There are several classes of blood pressure- lowering specifics, including diuretics, ACE impediments, calcium channel blockers, and beta- blockers. The drug specified will depend on colorful factors, including the case's age, the inflexibility of their hypertension, and any other medical conditions they may have.
Diuretics are specifics that help the body get relief of redundant fluid and swab through urine. They're frequently specified as the first- line pharmacological

treatment for hypertension due to their effectiveness and low cost. Examples of diuretics include hydrochlorothiazide and chlorthalidone.

ACE impediments work by relaxing blood vessels, which helps to lower blood pressure. Examples of ACE impediments include lisinopril and enalapril. Calcium channel blockers also work by relaxing blood vessels and can be useful in treating hypertension. Some examples of calcium channel blockers include amlodipine and diltiazem. Beta- blockers are specifics that reduce the heart's workload, which lowers blood pressure. They're frequently used in combination with other specifics to control hypertension. Examples of beta- blockers include atenolol and metoprolol. In addition to specifics and life changes, some cases with severe hypertension may bear further invasive treatments, similar as surgery or implantable blood pressure monitoring bias.

These treatments are generally reserved for cases with resistant hypertension, which is defined as high blood pressure that can not be controlled with drugs. One illustration of an invasive treatment for hypertension is renal denervation.

Renal denervation involves using radiofrequency energy to damage the renal jitters that control blood pressure.

This can help to reduce blood pressure situations in cases with resistant hypertension. Implantable blood pressure monitoring bias may also be used in cases with severe hypertension. These biases are generally placed inside the body, near the blood vessels, and can continuously cover blood pressure situations.

By covering blood pressure more nearly, croakers can acclimate specifics more precisely to ensure that cases' blood pressure situations remain in a healthy range. In conclusion, high blood pressure is a common medical condition that can lead to serious health complications if left undressed. Fortunately, multitudinous treatment options are available for hypertension, including life changes, specifics, and more invasive treatments similar to surgery. Working with your healthcare professional, you can find the right treatment plan to help control your blood pressure and reduce your pitfalls of long- term health complications.

FOOD AND FRUIT THAT HELPS TO REDUCE HIGH BLOOD PRESSURE

The first food group that can help in reducing high blood pressure is lush foliage. lush foliage analogous to spinach, collard foliage, and kale are high in potassium, which can help reduce the quantum of sodium in the body. Sodium is a mineral that is generally set up in hearties and is known to increase blood pressure.

A study conducted by the American Heart Association set up that consuming lush foliage was linked to a significant drop in blood pressure and a lower trouble of cardiovascular complaint. It's recommended to consume at least one serving of lush foliage daily to reduce high blood pressure. Another food group that can help in reducing high blood pressure is berries. Berries analogous to blueberries, snorts, and strawberries are rich in antioxidants, which can help reduce inflammation and improve overall cardiovascular health.

A study conducted by the American Journal of Clinical Nutrition set up that consuming berries daily was linked to a significant reduction in blood pressure and a lower trouble of heart complaint. It's recommended to consume at least one serving of berries daily to reduce high blood pressure. Fruits are also an important part of reducing high blood pressure. Apples are one of the most recommended fruits to reduce high blood pressure. Apples are high in fiber, which can help reduce cholesterol situations in the blood. A study conducted by the British Medical Journal set up that consuming apples daily was linked to a significant drop in blood pressure and a lower trouble of stroke. It's recommended to consume at least one serving of apples daily to reduce high blood pressure. Another fruit that can help in reducing high blood pressure is bananas. Bananas are high in potassium, which can help reduce the quantum of sodium in the body.

A study conducted by the American Heart Association set up that consuming bananas daily was linked to a significant drop in blood pressure and a lower trouble of cardiovascular complaint. It's recommended to consume at least one serving of bananas daily to reduce high blood pressure. In addition to fruits and vegetables, there are other foods that can help in reducing high blood pressure. One of these foods is adipose fish. Adipose fish analogous as salmon, mackerel, and sardines are high in omega- 3 adipose acids, which can help reduce inflammation and improve cardiovascular health.

A study conducted by the American Heart Association set up that consuming adipose fish weekly was linked to a significant drop in blood pressure and a lower trouble of heart complaint. It's recommended to consume at least two servings of adipose fish daily to reduce high blood pressure.

Another food that can help in reducing high blood pressure is garlic. Garlic has been used thousands of times for its medicinal parcels. Garlic is rich in allicin, a conflation that has been shown to reduce blood pressure and improve overall cardiovascular health. A study conducted by the Cochrane Database of regular Reviews set up that consuming garlic domestic was linked to a significant drop in blood pressure. It's recommended to consume at least one clove of garlic daily to reduce high blood pressure.

In conclusion, high blood pressure is a common medical condition that can lead to serious health complications. Fortunately, making changes to one's diet can have a significant impact on reducing high blood pressure.

Foods analogous to lush foliage, berries, apples, bananas, adipose fish, and garlic all have salutary parcels that can help reduce blood pressure and improve overall cardiovascular health. It's recommended to consume a variety of these foods daily to reduce high blood pressure.

EXERCISE FOR HIGH BLOOD PRESSURE

Blood Pressure Staying Active and Healthy High blood pressure, also known as hypertension, is a common condition that affects millions of people around the world. It occurs when the force of the blood pushing against the walls of the blood vessels is constantly too high. This can lead to serious health problems, analogous to heart complaints, stroke, and order failure. Fortunately, there are multitudinous life changes that people can make to help lower their blood pressure, with exercise being one of the most effective. This essay will explore the benefits of exercise for high blood pressure and give practical advice on staying active and healthy. originally, it's important to understand the mechanisms by which exercise can lower blood pressure. Regular physical exertion helps to strengthen the heart, making it more effective at pumping blood, and also improves the plainness of the blood vessels, allowing them to dilate and contract more fluently. This can lead to a drop in resistance to blood inflow and a consequent reduction in blood pressure. Likewise, exercise can also help to reduce stress and anxiety, which are common threat factors for hypertension.

There are numerous different types of exercise that can be salutary for those with high blood pressure. Aerobic exercise, similar as brisk walking, running, cycling, or swimming, is particularly effective at lowering blood pressure. Experts recommend at least 150 twinkles of moderate- intensity aerobic exercise per week, or 75 twinkles of vigorous- intensity exercise, spread out over several sessions. Strength training exercises, similar to toning or resistance band exercises, can also be helpful, as they can make muscles and ameliorate overall body composition.

Eventually, inflexibility and balance exercises, similar as yoga or Pilates, can help to ameliorate posture, reduce stress, and help cascade in aged grown-ups. When starting an exercise program, it's important to consult with a healthcare professional to insure that it's safe and applicable for your individual requirements and fitness position. People with high blood pressure or other health conditions may need to start with lower- intensity exercise and gradually increase the duration and intensity over time.

It's also important to choose conditioning that are pleasurable and sustainable, similar as walking with musketeers or taking a cotillion class, in order to stick to a regular exercise routine. Another important consideration for those with high blood pressure is to cover their blood pressure ahead and after exercise.

It's recommended to check blood pressure at least 30 twinkles before exercising, and again within 30 twinkles after finishing. This can help to ensure that the exercise program is having a positive effect on blood pressure and that any implicit negative goods, similar to post-exercise hypotension, are minimized.

It's also important to stay doused during and after exercise, particularly during hot rainfall or violent exercise, in order to maintain proper blood volume and help dehumidification.

In addition to physical exercise, there are numerous other life changes that can help to lower blood pressure.

These include eating a healthy diet that's low in sodium and high in fruits, vegetables, and whole grains;

maintaining a healthy weight; quitting smoking; reducing alcohol input; and managing stress through ways similar as deep breathing, contemplation, or awareness.

By incorporating these strategies into a comprehensive life approach, individualities with high blood pressure can significantly reduce their threat of complications and ameliorate their quality of life. To conclude, exercise is an important tool for managing high blood pressure and reducing the threat of affiliated health complications. Through regular physical exertion, individualities can ameliorate heart health, reduce stress, and ameliorate overall fitness. Still, it's important to approach exercise with caution, particularly for those with underpinning health conditions, and to incorporate other life changes for maximum benefit. By making healthy choices and staying active, individualities with high blood pressure can achieve a better quality of life and reduce their threat of serious health problems.

Citations

1.precludingInfections.   https//www.cdc.gov/infection control/prevent- infections/prevention.html

2. World Health Organization.(2017, January). Health Topics   AntibioticResistance. https//www.who.int/newsroom/fact-sheets/detail/antibioti c- resistance.